DEFEATING CELIAC DISEASE WITH EXPERT GUIDANCE

Ultimate Solution Handbook For Patients, Guardians Or Family To Understand, Manage, Treat, Prevent, Reverse Symptoms And Live Well

DR. POTTER WHITLEY

Copyright © 2023 by Dr. Potter Whitley

All rights reserved. Except for brief quotations included in critical reviews and certain other noncommercial uses allowed by copyright law, no part of this publication may be reproduced, distributed, or transmitted in any form or by any means, including photocopying, recording, or other electronic or mechanical methods, without the publisher's prior written permission.

DISCLAIMER:

This book's contents are meant to be used solely for informative purposes. The information should not be used as a replacement for expert medical advice, diagnosis, or care.

The information contained in this book is accurate and reliable, having been verified by the author to the best of his ability. Nevertheless, the author disclaims all express and implied representations and warranties regarding the availability, correctness, appropriateness, completeness, and reliability of the material provided here. You bear full responsibility for any reliance you may have on such material.

For informational purposes, this book may make reference to or mention of certain people, things, websites, organizations, or other names. The author has no connection to, endorsement from, or recommendation for these organizations. The author's approval or validation is not implied by the inclusion of these references.

Any direct, indirect, incidental, special, or consequential damages resulting from using or not being able to use the material in this book are not covered by the author's liability policy. For medical advice and counsel particular to their circumstances, readers are advised to check with experienced healthcare specialists.

The content, materials, and information in this book are subject to change at any time without prior notice, at the author's discretion. The text may contain errors or omissions for which the author is not responsible.

By reading this book, you understand and accept the conditions of this disclaimer.

THE REASON BEHIND THIS BOOK

This book "Defeating Celiac Disease With Expert Guidance" is an invaluable resource for anyone attempting to navigate the intricacies of celiac disease. This book's exhaustive investigation starts with a close analysis of the ailment, giving readers a strong basis on which to grasp its subtleties. The first few chapters provide an essential foundation of knowledge, from causes and risk factors to the disease's significant effects on the body, allowing readers to gain a better understanding of celiac disease.

This work is notable for its thorough examination of the gluten relationship. The nuances of gluten, its sources, and the hidden risks present in common items are explored in detail for readers. The writers examine how gluten affects people with celiac disease, discussing the difficulties caused by cross-contamination and giving readers useful advice on how to lead a successful gluten-free lifestyle.

It might be difficult to adjust to a gluten-free lifestyle, but this book provides professional advice to make it easier. For anyone starting a gluten-free journey, this book serves as a helpful culinary guide, including everything from practical cooking techniques and recipes to help interpret food labels. Additionally, it broadens its scope to include safe dining situations, guaranteeing that people with Celiac disease can continue to enjoy a healthy, balanced diet.

This book's emphasis on working together with medical professionals is one of its special qualities. It clarifies the roles of dietitians, nutritionists, gastroenterologists, and mental health specialists in managing celiac disease, emphasizing the value of a multidisciplinary approach. This all-encompassing strategy guarantees that readers will have a comprehensive understanding of their health journey.

Beyond the fundamentals, this book discusses drugs and therapies, especially for celiac disease. It provides a perceptive synopsis, addressing the function of vitamins, enzymes, and prospective therapies in the future. This book addresses the many needs of kids, teens, adults, and senior citizens dealing with the difficulties of celiac disease by going over management techniques for various life phases.

Additionally, this book sheds light on how Celiac Disease intersects with other medical disorders, highlighting the significance of managing coexisting conditions and their effects on mental health. Additionally, the significance of genetics is discussed and recommendations for counseling, family screening, and genetic predisposition are made.

In keeping with its mission of empowering people, this book informs readers of the most recent findings and advancements in the field of celiac disease research. In addition to outlining the status of research as it stands today, it also looks at exciting developments and discoveries that could inspire readers to take part in clinical trials.

This book emphasizes the need for activism and community support, going beyond personal adventures. It provides advice on how to raise awareness, get involved in support networks, and lobby lawmakers for legislation that will improve the lives of people with celiac disease in general.

This book ends with methods for living a life beyond celiac disease, a thunderous crescendo. It presents a clear picture of a happy and healthy existence outside the limitations of the disease, honors success stories, and gives hope for the future. This book is an important resource for anyone hoping to overcome celiac disease and live a vibrant, healthy life since it is a beacon of knowledge and support.

TABLE OF CONTENTS

CHAPTER ONE 12

UNDERSTANDING CELIAC DISEASE 12

OVERVIEW OF CELIAC DISEASE: 12

REASONS AND DANGER FACTORS: 13

SYMPTOMS AND INDICATIONS: 14

EVALUATION AND DIAGNOSIS: 16

EFFECT ON THE HUMAN BODY: 18

CHAPTER TWO 22

THE RELATIONSHIP WITH GLUTEN 22

INVESTIGATING GLUTEN AND ITS ORIGINS: 22

HOW CELIAC PATIENTS ARE AFFECTED BY GLUTEN: 23

UNCOVERED GLUTEN IN COMMON PRODUCTS: 24

GLUTEN CROSS-CONTAMINATION: 25

CHAPTER THREE 28

MANAGING A GLUTEN-FREE WAY OF LIVING 28

CHANGING YOUR DIET TO A GLUTEN-FREE ONE: 28

EFFECTIVE FOOD LABEL READING: 29

GLUTEN-FREE RECIPES AND COOKING ADVICE: 31

SAFE DINING OUT: 32

CHAPTER FOUR 34

PROFESSIONAL ADVICE FOR MANAGING CELIAC DISEASE 34

THE ROLE OF MEDICAL EXPERTS IN THE MANAGEMENT OF CELIAC DISEASE: 34

NUTRITIONISTS AND DIETITIANS IN CELIAC DISEASE CARE: 36

WORKING IN PARTNERSHIP WITH GASTROENTEROLOGISTS: 37

ASSISTANCE FROM MENTAL HEALTH SPECIALISTS: 39

CHAPTER FIVE 42

DRUGS AND THERAPIES 42
SYNOPSIS OF DRUGS PARTICULAR TO CELIAC DISEASE: 42
FUNCTION OF SUPPLEMENTS AND ENZYMES: 44
POSSIBLE COURSE OF TREATMENTS: 45

CHAPTER SIX 48

MANAGING CELIAC IN DIFFERENT LIFE STAGES 48
CELIAC DISEASE IN CHILDREN: 48
TEENS AND ADOLESCENTS: 49
GLUTEN INTOLERANCE IN THE ADULT: 50
SENIORS AND CELIAC DISEASE: 51

CHAPTER SEVEN 52

OTHER HEALTH CONDITIONS AND CELIAC DISEASE 52
FREQUENTLY OCCURRING CONDITIONS: 52
HANDLING SEVERAL HEALTH CONCERNS: 53
INFLUENCE ON MENTAL WELL-BEING: 55

CHAPTER EIGHT 58

GENETIC FACTORS ASSOCIATED WITH CELIAC DISEASE 58
GENETIC PREDISPOSITION AND CELIAC DISEASE: 58
FAMILY SCREENING AND GENETIC COUNSELING: 60

CHAPTER NINE 62

RESEARCH AND DEVELOPMENTS TO KEEP YOU INFORMED 62
RESEARCH ON CELIAC DISEASE AS OF RIGHT NOW: 62
PROSPECTIVE DEVELOPMENTS AND INNOVATIONS: 64

Taking Part in Clinical Research: 67

CHAPTER TEN..70

COMMUNITY SUPPORT AND ADVOCACY.......................70
Raising Awareness of Celiac Disease:...........................70
Joining Support Groups for Celiacs: 71
Promoting Changes in Policy:.....................................72

CHAPTER ELEVEN 76

OVERCOMING CELIAC DISEASE TO SUCCEED 76
Techniques for Living a Happy and Healthful Life 76
Honoring Achievements 78
Outlook for Celiac Patients in the Future.....................79

CHAPTER ONE

UNDERSTANDING CELIAC DISEASE
Overview of Celiac Disease:

In people with celiac disease, a long-term autoimmune illness, eating gluten damages the small intestine. In those with celiac disease, gluten—a protein present in wheat, barley, and rye—sets off an immunological reaction that damages the lining of the small intestine and causes inflammation. Nutrient absorption is hampered by this damage, which can result in a variety of symptoms and even more serious issues. Celiac disease necessitates a rigorous gluten-free diet and is a lifelong condition, unlike wheat allergies or gluten sensitivity.

Any age can be affected by celiac disease, and in recent years, its prevalence has increased. There is a significant hereditary component to the illness, even though its precise etiology is unknown. Those who have a family history of celiac disease are more likely to get the illness. Furthermore, the timing of introducing gluten into an infant's diet and other environmental factors, like illnesses throughout early childhood, may contribute to the disease's onset.

Celiac disease is an autoimmune illness in which eating gluten causes the immune system to wrongly attack the body's tissues. The typical damage observed in the small intestine can be attributed to a series of events that are set off by this immune response. It is essential to comprehend the complexities of the immune system's involvement in celiac disease to create therapies and treatments that work.

Reasons and Danger Factors:

The etiology of celiac disease is complex, involving both environmental and genetic factors. The human leukocyte antigen (HLA) genotypes HLA-DQ2 and HLA-DQ8, in particular, are the main genetic factors linked to celiac disease. When exposed to gluten, those who carry certain genetic markers are more likely to develop celiac disease.

Environmental variables play a role in the development of celiac disease in addition to hereditary factors. Several factors have been linked, including the timing of introducing gluten into a baby's diet and the frequency of gastrointestinal illnesses in the early years of life. Moreover, autoimmune thyroid problems and type 1 diabetes are among the illnesses that frequently occur with celiac disease, suggesting a complicated interaction between several autoimmune conditions.

Acknowledging the various risk factors linked to celiac disease is crucial to pinpoint those who might be more vulnerable and put preventative measures in place. Furthermore, by comprehending how genetics and environment interact, treatment strategies that target immune response modulation and celiac disease prevention in at-risk individuals may be able to be targeted.

Symptoms and Indications:

There is a large range of signs and symptoms associated with celiac disease, which can often make diagnosis difficult. Individuals may have little or no symptoms at all, and symptoms might vary widely throughout people. Gastrointestinal problems include diarrhea, bloating, stomach discomfort, and weight loss are typical symptoms. Celiac disease, however, can also cause non-gastrointestinal symptoms like weariness, joint discomfort, and skin rashes in addition to its digestive symptoms.

Celiac illness can affect a child's growth and development, delaying puberty and causing stunted growth. Understanding the many clinical manifestations of celiac disease is essential for healthcare professionals to promote early diagnosis and treatment. Furthermore, the range of symptoms emphasizes how crucial it is to rule out celiac disease in a broad differential diagnosis, particularly in cases when patients present with complaints that don't seem to be connected.

In addition to the obvious physical symptoms, celiac disease can have a major effect on general well-being and mental health. Suffering from a chronic illness that necessitates close dietary compliance can exacerbate anxiety and despair. Thus, to diagnose celiac disease patients promptly and accurately and improve their quality of life and management, medical personnel must have a thorough awareness of the condition's indications and symptoms.

Evaluation and Diagnosis:

For appropriate therapy for celiac disease to begin and long-term problems to be avoided, an accurate and fast diagnosis is essential. Usually, a mix of clinical assessment, serological testing, and confirmation tests like endoscopy with biopsy are used in the diagnosis process. Specific antibodies linked to celiac disease, such as anti-tissue transglutaminase (tTG) and anti-endomysial antibodies (EMA), are measured by serological testing. Increased concentrations of these antibodies may signify the existence of an immunological reaction provoked by gluten.

Even though serological testing are useful screening method, small intestinal specimens taken during endoscopy frequently need to be histologically examined to reach a conclusive diagnosis. Intraepithelial lymphocytosis, crypt hyperplasia, and villous atrophy are typical histological findings. A thorough grasp of the scope and severity of the disease is possible through the combination of serological and histological evaluations.

Medical professionals must take into account the constraints and possible hazards associated with diagnosis, such as the requirement for continuous gluten consumption to obtain reliable test results. Furthermore, being aware of illnesses that can mimic celiac disease—like non-celiac gluten sensitivity—helps ensure proper management techniques and prevents misdiagnoses.

New biomarkers and non-invasive testing techniques are being researched as part of the constantly changing field of celiac disease diagnostics. The ultimate goal of these developments is to help people with celiac disease by enabling early detection and care. They also seek to increase accessibility to testing, optimize the diagnostic process, and increase diagnostic accuracy.

Effect on the Human Body:

The body is profoundly affected by celiac disease, which affects several organ systems and has a variety of short- and long-term effects. The small intestine is the main area affected, as poor nutrient absorption is caused by villous atrophy and persistent inflammation. Many dietary deficits, such as those in iron, calcium, vitamin D, and B vitamins, can result from this malabsorption.

Celiac disease can cause symptoms that are not limited to the small intestine; it can also affect the pancreas, liver, and gallbladder. Elevated liver enzymes and autoimmune hepatitis are examples of liver disorders that highlight the disease's systemic character. Furthermore, there may be a higher chance of problems including pancreatitis and gallstones in people with celiac disease.

Apart from the effects on the gastrointestinal system, celiac disease is linked to an increased likelihood of acquiring further autoimmune disorders. These can include rheumatoid arthritis, type 1 diabetes, and autoimmune thyroid diseases. The connection between celiac disease and other autoimmune diseases highlights the intricate interactions occurring within the immune system and the necessity of treating autoimmune diseases holistically.

The immediate gastrointestinal and immunological complications of celiac disease are not the only long-term implications of untreated or inadequately managed disease. Celiac disease patients may be more susceptible to osteoporosis, infertility, and some malignancies, including lymphomas. Understanding and treating the systemic effects of celiac disease is crucial to developing tailored, all-encompassing management plans that put the patient's general health and well-being first.

In conclusion, it is critical for medical experts, those who are afflicted with the illness, and the general public to comprehend the complex facets of celiac disease, from its origins and introduction to its wide range of symptoms, diagnostic techniques, and systemic effects on the body. This thorough understanding serves as the cornerstone for management decisions that are well-informed, continuous research targeted at expanding our understanding of celiac disease, and better results for people who suffer from it.

CHAPTER TWO

THE RELATIONSHIP WITH GLUTEN
Investigating Gluten and Its Origins:

The complex protein combination known as gluten is present in wheat and kindred cereals and is essential to the texture and elasticity of a wide range of food products. Those with celiac disease need to understand its causes. The main offenders are wheat, barley, and rye; gluten is also present in derivatives like malt and semolina. This protein can be found in surprising areas, such as soups, sauces, and even some drugs. It is not just found in bread and pasta. Gluten is widely used in the modern diet as a stabilizing or thickening ingredient by manufacturers.

Furthermore, gluten isn't just found in food. It also occurs in playdough, cosmetics, and several pharmaceuticals, which presents further difficulties for people who have celiac disease. It becomes crucial to thoroughly investigate gluten sources for both patients and medical professionals.

A thorough understanding of these resources enables people to make knowledgeable decisions regarding their food and way of life, which promotes improved celiac disease management.

How Celiac Patients Are Affected by Gluten:

A comprehensive grasp of the complex interactions between gluten and celiac disease patients is necessary for successful treatment. Gluten consumption causes an immunological reaction in people with celiac disease, an autoimmune condition that affects the lining of the small intestine. This damage reduces the body's ability to absorb nutrients and can cause a variety of symptoms, such as joint pain, exhaustion, and gastrointestinal problems.

Gluten is more than simply an annoyance for those with celiac disease; it's a trigger for a convoluted series of events in the body. Severe side effects from long-term gluten intake can include osteoporosis, malnutrition, and an elevated chance of developing further autoimmune diseases. Because the disorder is persistent, the effects sometimes extend beyond physical health and damage mental well-being. Thus, understanding the significant impacts of gluten on individuals with celiac disease is essential to creating treatment and preventative plans that work.

Uncovered Gluten in Common Products:

There's more to navigating the world of gluten-containing food than just figuring out the obvious offenders, like bread and spaghetti. For those suffering from celiac disease, hidden sources of gluten can be particularly problematic because this protein can be found in many commonplace items and processed foods without obvious labeling. Carefully reading labels is essential because gluten can be found in sauces, condiments, and even seemingly harmless products like vitamins.

The need for increased caution is highlighted by the misleading nature of concealed gluten. Encouraging celiac patients to identify hidden gluten in ingredient lists and understand how to interpret them will enable them to make decisions that respect their dietary restrictions. Furthermore, having this knowledge helps cultivate a sense of autonomy and control, both of which are essential for successfully managing celiac disease on a day-to-day basis.

Gluten cross-contamination:

For people with celiac disease, the threat of gluten cross-contamination looms large, complicating already difficult dietary choices. When gluten-free foods come into touch with surfaces, utensils, or goods that have come into contact with gluten-containing things, it's known as cross-contamination. This can occur in communal kitchens, dining establishments, or even during food preparation.

Cross-contamination prevention necessitates a multipronged strategy. Both individuals and restaurants need to be proactive in conveying dietary needs. Strict processes must be implemented. It also becomes essential to designate certain areas in communal kitchens and residences for gluten-free cooking. To protect their health and maintain a completely gluten-free lifestyle, celiac sufferers must comprehend the subtleties of gluten cross-contamination.

CHAPTER THREE

MANAGING A GLUTEN-FREE WAY OF LIVING
Changing Your Diet to a Gluten-Free One:

For those with celiac disease, making the switch to a gluten-free diet can be a big adjustment. It entails removing grains like wheat, barley, and rye that contain gluten from one's diet. Making the switch involves more than just replacing standard items with gluten-free alternatives. It necessitates a deep comprehension of food ingredients and knowledge of any potential gluten-containing hidden sources.

The education component of this shift is crucial. Patients must familiarize themselves with naturally gluten-free meals and educate themselves about gluten-free substitutes. This includes knowing which grains, such as rice and quinoa, are gluten-free as well as the range of gluten-free flours that can be used in baking.

People also need to be mindful of cross-contamination, making sure that appliances, kitchen surfaces, and utensils are all well-cleansed to avoid unintentionally coming into contact with gluten.

Making the switch to a gluten-free diet also requires careful consideration of social and emotional factors. Online and offline support groups can offer insightful information and emotional support throughout this process. Interacting with people who have effectively transitioned to a gluten-free lifestyle can provide helpful advice and motivation. It's important to look at this change as a chance to experiment with other foods and cooking methods rather than concentrating just on the restrictions associated with a gluten-free diet.

Effective Food Label Reading:

The key to successful gluten-free living is being able to interpret food labels. Because gluten can appear under many names in ingredient lists, people with celiac disease must learn how to read labels.

It's essential to comprehend words like malt extract, hydrolyzed vegetable protein, and modified food starch when attempting to detect possible gluten sources in packaged meals.

Furthermore, regional variations in the requirements for gluten-free labeling add yet another level of complexity. To guarantee adherence to set criteria, it's a good idea to search for items verified by respectable gluten-free certifying organizations. In addition to gluten, people need to be aware of other allergies that might be present in processed foods.

Food makers may reformulate their products, and ingredients may vary over time, thus constant observation is necessary. A safe and nutritious gluten-free diet can be maintained by keeping up with the most recent changes to the laws governing gluten-free labeling and seeking advice from medical experts.

Gluten-Free Recipes and Cooking Advice:

Adopting a gluten-free lifestyle entails learning how to cook without gluten in addition to avoiding it. Trying different flours, including almond flour, coconut flour, and chickpea flour, offers you a whole new range of options for making tasty and secure meals. Cooking without gluten is a creative activity that inspires people to experiment with different ingredients and culinary traditions.

To achieve the proper texture and flavor in homemade gluten-free items, one must understand the science of gluten-free baking. For instance, adding xanthan gum or guar gum can replicate the gluten's binding qualities and give baked goods structure. It also improves the whole dining experience to learn how to combine flavors and textures without depending on gluten-containing products.

Having a library of gluten-free meals at hand is crucial to keeping a diet varied. A plethora of inspiration may be found in cookbooks, online resources, and cooking classes specifically designed for gluten-free living. People may find a variety of culinary treats that meet their dietary requirements, from rich sweets to gluten-free pasta dishes.

Safe Dining Out:

For those with celiac disease, eating out might be difficult, but it is possible to enjoy restaurant meals safely with careful planning and discussion. The first step is to pick eateries that are aware of gluten-free policies. Businesses that cater to people with celiac disease by providing gluten-free menus or properly labeling gluten-free options show their dedication to this community.

It's critical to communicate effectively with restaurant employees. Cross-contamination can be reduced by telling servers about dietary restrictions and thoroughly inquiring about food preparation techniques. The significance of avoiding even minute levels of gluten must be emphasized to avoid negative health impacts.

It's important to know where hidden gluten is typically found in restaurant food. It's important to ask about sauces, marinades, and thickeners when placing an order because these items frequently include gluten. Some people find it beneficial to stick to naturally gluten-free cuisines, such as Thai or Mexican, which typically feature rice or corn-based dishes.

In summary, living a gluten-free lifestyle requires a variety of skills, from learning how to cook gluten-free food to securely navigating restaurant menus. It also requires a gradual shift to a gluten-free diet and accurate food label reading. People with celiac disease can manage their condition and live on a gluten-free diet by seeking education, and support, and being open to trying new foods.

CHAPTER FOUR

PROFESSIONAL ADVICE FOR MANAGING CELIAC DISEASE
The Role of Medical Experts in the Management of Celiac Disease:

The engagement of medical specialists is crucial in the holistic approach to managing celiac disease. First off, gastroenterologists are frequently needed for the first diagnosis of celiac disease. These experts have the necessary training to identify the symptoms, carry out pertinent diagnostic procedures, and establish the autoimmune disorder's existence. Their ability to diagnose quickly and accurately guarantees that those with celiac disease are identified, which paves the way for efficient treatment.

After a diagnosis, continuing medical monitoring is essential for managing the complications associated with celiac disease. Frequent check-ups with medical professionals allow for condition monitoring, which guarantees rapid resolution of any new problems or difficulties. Medical practitioners can help people understand the possible side effects of celiac disease, such as dietary deficits or the possibility of developing other autoimmune conditions.

Medical experts are also necessary in creating a customized treatment strategy. This includes counseling on lifestyle modifications in addition to writing prescriptions for required drugs. For example, people with Celiac disease frequently need to be cautious about their exposure to gluten, and doctors are essential in helping patients understand dietary choices and possible hidden sources of gluten.

In conclusion, medical experts play a critical role in managing celiac disease at every step, from diagnosis to continued treatment. Their knowledge guarantees precise identification, ongoing observation, and the creation of an all-encompassing treatment plan customized to meet the specific requirements of every patient.

Nutritionists and Dietitians in Celiac Disease Care:

A person with celiac disease must follow a strict diet to maintain good health, and dietitians and nutritionists are invaluable in this regard. These experts give individualized guidance to address each patient's specific dietary requirements and issues because they have a sophisticated understanding of the intricate interactions between nutrition and celiac disease.

Helping people follow a strict gluten-free diet is one of the main duties of dietitians and nutritionists. This entails not just removing apparent gluten sources but also deciphering food labels and finding gluten that may be concealed in a variety of items. Dietitians are essential in helping patients understand safe, substitute food options so that their nutritional demands can be satisfied even with the dietary limitations brought on by celiac disease.

Dietitians address various nutritional deficiencies that may emerge in persons with Celiac disease, in addition to gluten avoidance. Together, they and the patients create a balanced meal plan that makes up for any deficiencies in vitamins, minerals, or other necessary components. This preventive measure lowers the chance of subsequent problems linked to malnutrition while also promoting general health.

To sum up, the knowledge that dietitians and nutritionists possess is invaluable when it comes to celiac care. Their advice enables people to make knowledgeable food decisions, which supports not only the efficient management of celiac disease but also the preservation of ideal nutritional status and general health.

Working in Partnership with Gastroenterologists:

Effective care for celiac disease is largely dependent on cooperation between patients with the autoimmune condition and gastroenterologists. As medical professionals who specialize in the digestive tract, gastroenterologists offer a breadth of expertise that is essential for the identification, management, and continuous care of celiac disease.

Accurately diagnosing celiac disease is the first step in the cooperation. Endoscopic procedures and blood tests are among the tests and evaluations that gastroenterologists are qualified to do to confirm the diagnosis of the condition. To guarantee that patients receive the right care and interventions customized to their unique case of celiac disease, this diagnostic precision is essential.

The continued collaboration with gastroenterologists becomes crucial after diagnosis. Frequent examinations and consultations offer a forum for tracking the development of celiac disease, evaluating the efficacy of treatment, and treating any new issues. To treat related disorders like irritable bowel syndrome or inflammatory bowel disease, which can coexist with celiac disease, gastroenterologists are essential.

Gastroenterologists also provide insightful information about the wider effects of celiac disease. They offer advice on possible long-term hazards, such as the emergence of further autoimmune diseases or difficulties brought on by dietary deficiencies. This all-encompassing strategy guarantees that patients receive prompt medical care along with proactive advice to improve their general health.

In conclusion, managing celiac disease involves a dynamic and continuing partnership with gastroenterologists. Their ongoing involvement and specialized knowledge make a substantial contribution to the general health of patients with celiac disease as well as to correct diagnosis and individualized treatment regimens.

Assistance from Mental Health Specialists:

Celiac disease affects people's mental and emotional health in addition to their physical health. The psychological ramifications of managing a chronic illness such as celiac disease can be complex, necessitating the assistance and knowledge of mental health specialists. Therapists, counselors, and psychologists are essential in helping people deal with the emotional difficulties that come with having celiac disease.

People may feel a variety of emotions after receiving a diagnosis, such as anger, fear, or even sadness at what they perceive to be a loss of culinary freedom. Mental health practitioners offer a secure and encouraging environment for people to communicate these feelings, assisting them in coping with the psychological effects of celiac disease. To promote resilience and ease the transition to a gluten-free lifestyle, this emotional support is essential.

Additionally, mental health specialists help people create coping mechanisms for the particular stresses involved in managing a chronic illness. This could entail addressing worries about social settings, including eating out or going to events where a lot of gluten-containing food is served. Mental health specialists help patients to lead fulfilled lives despite the challenges given by Celiac disease by providing them with efficient coping methods.

When people struggle to follow a gluten-free diet or experience issues with their body image, mental health providers provide specialized interventions. To promote a comprehensive approach to well-being, they collaborate with patients to investigate and treat any underlying psychological issues that can impede efficient disease management.

In summary, getting help from mental health specialists is essential to managing celiac disease. Mental health experts play a vital role in improving the overall quality of life for those with Celiac disease by addressing the emotional and psychological aspects of living with this condition.

CHAPTER FIVE

DRUGS AND THERAPIES
Synopsis of Drugs Particular to Celiac Disease:

The autoimmune condition celiac disease, which is brought on by eating gluten, needs to be carefully managed. Although the main course of treatment is still a strict gluten-free diet, several drugs can be very helpful in reducing symptoms and encouraging intestinal healing. Corticosteroids are one such drug that is used to treat severe small intestinal irritation. These drugs may be especially helpful for people who are dealing with acute problems or symptoms. However, because of possible adverse consequences, its long-term usage is frequently restricted.

Immunosuppressants are another family of drugs that have demonstrated potential in the treatment of celiac disease. By inhibiting the immune system's reaction to gluten, these medications lessen inflammation and small intestinal damage.

They are usually only used in situations when other therapies are deemed insufficient, and close observation is necessary to reduce any possible hazards.

Furthermore, studies on drugs that specifically target immunological mechanisms implicated in the onset of celiac disease are being conducted. One such medication is larazotide acetate, which works by keeping the tight connections in the intestine from leaking and, as a result, lowering the body's reaction to gluten. Positive outcomes from clinical trials give optimism for a future with more specialized and efficient treatment options.

It is important to stress that, even with these advancements, drugs are not a stand-alone treatment for celiac disease. The mainstay of care continues to be a gluten-free diet and to maximize results, prescription drugs are frequently combined with dietary changes.

Function of Supplements and Enzymes:

Supplements and enzymes are essential in the treatment of celiac disease, offering extra assistance to those overcoming the difficulties associated with a gluten-free diet. Tissue transglutaminase is one important enzyme under investigation since it is essential to the autoimmune reaction brought on by gluten. Studies have looked into the possibility of creating drugs that specifically target this enzyme to lessen intestinal damage and the immunological response. Even if these advancements show promise, research on them is still in its early phases.

When it comes to vitamins, people with celiac disease frequently worry about nutritional deficits. Deficiencies in vitamins and minerals, including iron, calcium, and vitamin D, can result from malabsorption problems in the damaged intestine. Therefore, it is frequently advised to take supplements to fill in these nutritional deficiencies and promote general health. To ascertain their unique needs, people must, therefore, consult closely with healthcare providers because taking too many supplements can also be dangerous.

Probiotics have also drawn interest because of their possible contribution to gut health promotion. Probiotics and celiac disease: A study is still being done, but some probiotic strains may help regulate immune response and enhance the function of the gut barrier. Under the supervision of a healthcare professional, adding probiotics to the treatment regimen may provide further assistance for those with celiac disease.

Possible Course of Treatments:

Treatment options for celiac disease are changing as a result of continuing research that is opening doors to possible new treatments. The creation of drugs that specifically target immunological mechanisms linked to the onset of the disease is one line of inquiry. For example, the ability of monoclonal antibodies to specifically suppress important elements of the immune response to gluten is being studied to potentially offer a more focused and successful treatment strategy.

Investigating the enzymes that break down gluten is another topic of study. Enzymes that can break down gluten molecules in the digestive tract and lessen the chance of inciting an immunological response are being researched. Although a gluten-free diet is not meant to be replaced by these enzymes, they might provide an extra degree of safety for those with celiac disease who might unintentionally ingest trace amounts of gluten.

Immunotherapy is seeing an increase in interest in desensitization techniques that try to rewire the immune system's reaction to gluten. Clinical trials are investigating the use of immune-modulating drugs in conjunction with gradual, controlled exposure to gluten. If effective, this strategy could completely change how celiac disease is managed by giving patients more food options.

In conclusion, continued research into specific drugs, enzymes, and immunotherapies bodes well for the treatment of celiac disease. Beyond the present focus on a strict gluten-free diet, these possible medicines may offer additional pathways for controlling celiac disease as they move through clinical trials and regulatory processes. To advance these cutting-edge strategies and enhance outcomes for those afflicted with this autoimmune illness, researchers, medical professionals, and people with celiac disease must continue to collaborate.

CHAPTER SIX

MANAGING CELIAC IN DIFFERENT LIFE STAGES
Celiac Disease in Children:

Given that children with celiac disease are frequently diagnosed at a young age, they present special challenges. During this period of life, the condition must be managed with a holistic approach that takes into account the child's emotional and physical health. The main emphasis is on following a rigorous gluten-free diet, which can be difficult for kids who might not grasp what their dietary restrictions mean. To create a supportive environment at home and educate their children about gluten-containing meals and alternatives, parents play a critical role.

Pediatricians and nutritionists are crucial partners in the treatment of celiac disease in children, even when it comes to dietary concerns. To guarantee healthy growth and development, routine examinations and nutritional status monitoring are essential. In addition, consulting a child psychologist or counselor can help address the possible psychological effects of having a chronic illness. Peer support groups can also assist kids in making connections with others going through comparable struggles, which can lessen feelings of loneliness and promote a sense of belonging.

Teens and Adolescents:

The treatment of celiac disease in children changes as they enter puberty and teenage years, taking into account their growing independence and social interactions. It gets harder to stick to a gluten-free diet because of social pressures, peer pressure, and the need for independence. Healthcare professionals must enable youth to make educated food decisions by stressing the long-term effects of non-compliance.

Friends, instructors, and school personnel should also get education regarding celiac disease in addition to the individual affected. To prevent feelings of isolation and encourage cooperation in the management of the disease, schools must foster an inclusive and understanding environment.

To ensure teens' safety and well-being, particularly in social circumstances, they must be encouraged to acquire appropriate communication skills regarding their dietary needs.

Gluten Intolerance in the Adult:

Throughout adulthood, managing celiac disease requires juggling several facets of life, such as relationships, work, and general well-being. Adults need to continue following a gluten-free diet be careful to read food labels and prevent cross-contamination. It's imperative to schedule routine check-ups with medical professionals to keep an eye out for any potential issues, like autoimmune diseases or nutritional deficiencies.

People who have celiac disease may need to speak out about their dietary needs at work and inform coworkers of the need to keep the workplace gluten-free. Developing a solid support system in both personal and professional spheres can be very helpful in managing celiac disease in maturity.

Seniors and celiac disease:

Seniors with celiac disease have special considerations because aging can bring on new health issues. While following a gluten-free diet is still essential, making food decisions may become more difficult due to things like altered digestive processes, less appetite, and dental problems. It becomes more crucial to regularly check for dietary deficits, bone health issues, and other age-related issues.

Seniors with celiac disease need social assistance more than anyone else since they may have more difficulty finding gluten-free foods and following dietary guidelines. Participating in community events and support groups can offer guidance and emotional support. Working together with medical specialists, such as dietitians and geriatricians, guarantees that the unique requirements of elderly people with celiac disease are fully met, enhancing general health and well-being.

CHAPTER SEVEN

OTHER HEALTH CONDITIONS AND CELIAC DISEASE
Frequently Occurring Conditions:

Gluten ingestion causes the autoimmune disease celiac disease, which frequently coexists with several other medical disorders. The most common correlation is with autoimmune diseases. Thyroid issues, rheumatoid arthritis, and type 1 diabetes are among the autoimmune diseases that people with celiac disease are more likely to have. This incidence raises the possibility that there is a genetic propensity shared by these conditions, underscoring the significance of careful medical monitoring for those with celiac disease.

Dermatitis herpetiformis (DH) is a skin manifestation of celiac disease and is another common comorbid ailment. The hallmark of DH is extremely painful, blistering skin lesions, which frequently point to underlying gluten sensitivity. Celiac disease has also been connected to neurological disorders such as epilepsy and peripheral neuropathy. These correlations underscore the systemic character of celiac disease, highlighting the necessity of comprehensive healthcare strategies that address possible problems impacting several organ systems in addition to gastrointestinal symptoms.

Moreover, disorders of the reproductive system might be linked to celiac disease. Untreated celiac disease increases the chance of miscarriage and can affect a woman's ability to conceive. Those who have celiac disease should be aware of these possible concomitant illnesses because early diagnosis and treatment can greatly enhance overall health outcomes.

Handling Several Health Concerns:

An interdisciplinary approach is necessary for managing various health conditions in the setting of celiac disease. Strict devotion to a gluten-free diet—removing the protein that sets off the autoimmune response—is the cornerstone of care.

This dietary adjustment is crucial for managing celiac disease as well as avoiding complications and co-occurring diseases.

It's essential to have regular medical monitoring to identify and quickly treat any new health problems. This entails working along with dermatologists, gastroenterologists, endocrinologists, and other experts as needed. The success of the gluten-free diet is tracked and any potential issues are identified with the aid of routine blood tests, imaging examinations, and clinical evaluations.

Because malabsorption of vital vitamins and minerals is prevalent, people with celiac disease benefit from dietary counseling in addition to medical therapy to make sure they receive enough nutrients. It could be advised to use dietary supplements to make up for some deficits and improve general health.

Another essential element of addressing the various health problems linked to celiac disease is psychosocial assistance.

People with chronic autoimmune conditions can benefit from support groups, therapy, and educational materials to help them deal with the difficulties of their disease.

When treating celiac disease and its concomitant disorders, a comprehensive strategy that takes into account mental and physical health aspects improves quality of life.

Influence on Mental Well-Being:

Beyond its clinical manifestations, celiac disease affects mental health, having an impact on general quality of life and emotional well-being. People with celiac disease often experience elevated levels of stress, anxiety, and depression due to the chronic nature of their condition and the requirement for a strict gluten-free diet.

The psychological load is increased by the need for constant attention to avoid gluten-containing foods, the possibility of social isolation brought on by dietary restrictions, and the uncertainty of having a chronic autoimmune disease. The emotional difficulties that people with celiac disease confront are further complicated by the diagnosis and treatment of comorbid diseases.

There is a reciprocal relationship between mental health and celiac disease. Inducing a vicious cycle of both physical and mental discomfort, stress and emotional factors can make gastrointestinal problems worse. As a result, providing comprehensive care for celiac disease requires addressing its psychosocial elements.

Counseling and support groups are examples of psychosocial support, which is essential for lessening the negative effects on mental health. Education materials that support resilience, stress reduction, and coping mechanisms are useful aids for those navigating the emotional challenges of celiac disease.

A more holistic approach is fostered by including mental health services in the treatment plan, which improves emotional well-being and raises the quality of life for people with celiac disease and its associated diseases.

CHAPTER EIGHT

GENETIC FACTORS ASSOCIATED WITH CELIAC DISEASE
Genetic Predisposition and Celiac Disease:

The autoimmune condition celiac disease, which is brought on by eating gluten, has long been known to have a significant hereditary component. Genetics plays a crucial part in celiac disease, as some genes greatly impact an individual's vulnerability to the illness.

The HLA-DQ2 and HLA-DQ8 genes, in particular, are part of the human leukocyte antigen (HLA) complex, which has been implicated in the development of celiac disease. When exposed to gluten, those with certain genetic variations are more likely to develop celiac disease.

90% of people with celiac disease have the HLA-DQ2 gene. This represents the majority of cases. In the meanwhile, the remaining instances are linked to the HLA-DQ8 gene. These genes encode essential immune system proteins, and variations in these genes lead to the aberrant immunological response observed in celiac disease. For those who have these genetic predispositions, eating gluten causes the small intestine's lining to be damaged by an immune response, which results in the symptoms that are specific to celiac disease.

Early diagnosis and care for celiac disease are contingent upon an understanding of the genetic variables linked to the condition. Genetic testing can detect those who are more susceptible, enabling preventative actions to be performed before the development of symptoms.

Furthermore, understanding the genetic underpinnings of celiac disease facilitates continued research attempts to create tailored treatments that target the underlying processes triggering the autoimmune reaction.

Family Screening And Genetic Counseling:

Family screening is essential for identifying persons at risk and putting preventive measures in place because celiac disease is inherited. It is critical to evaluate the risk for close family members when a diagnosis is made for one member of the family.

The HLA-DQ2 or HLA-DQ8 genes can be found by genetic screening, which can provide important information regarding a person's risk of developing celiac disease.

Family screening aims to stop the disease from progressing in those who are at risk as well as identify those who are afflicted. A gluten-free diet can be implemented before the onset of symptoms thanks to early detection through genetic testing, which may prevent the development of issues connected to celiac disease. In addition, it empowers families to make well-informed decisions on dietary modifications and lifestyle choices that promote the general well-being of impacted individuals.

A crucial part of the process of screening a family for celiac disease is genetic counseling. Genetic counselors offer thorough information to individuals and their families regarding the condition's genetic origin, the ramifications of positive test results, and the available preventive strategies. By enabling people to make knowledgeable decisions about their own and their family members' health, this counseling promotes a proactive approach to managing celiac disease in the context of the family.

To sum up, family screening along with genetic counseling and knowledge of the genetic variables influencing celiac propensity are essential to the holistic therapy of celiac disease. These methods support early diagnosis and intervention while also giving people and families the power to make decisions that will improve their health and general well-being.

CHAPTER NINE

RESEARCH AND DEVELOPMENTS TO KEEP YOU INFORMED
Research On Celiac Disease As Of Right Now:

Research into celiac disease, an autoimmune condition brought on by gluten ingestion, has advanced significantly in recent years. To create more potent diagnostic instruments and therapeutic strategies, researchers are diving deeper into comprehending the complex mechanisms behind the illness. The genetic component of celiac disease is a crucial field of research, with several genetic markers linked to a higher vulnerability being revealed by certain studies. This information helps with early detection and offers suggestions for preventative actions.

Furthermore, the various clinical manifestations of celiac disease that go beyond the traditional gastrointestinal symptoms are becoming more widely recognized.

To better understand the systemic aspect of celiac disease, researchers are looking into connections between the illness and several other ailments, including dermatitis herpetiformis and neurological diseases. This deeper comprehension is essential for prompt diagnosis and all-encompassing treatment plans.

Furthermore, technological developments have made it possible to use more precise and effective diagnostic techniques. The increased sophistication of serological tests, genetic testing, and intestinal biopsies has made it possible to diagnose celiac disease earlier and with more accuracy. Innovative imaging modalities such as capsule endoscopy provide non-invasive substitutes for determining the degree of intestinal injury. These advancements in diagnosis are critical to the timely identification of those who have celiac disease, which enables lifestyle modifications and treatments.

The involvement of the gut microbiota in celiac disease is another topic of research interest. There's growing evidence that the makeup of gut bacteria may have a role in the onset and course of the illness. Gaining insight into these complex relationships may pave the way for novel therapeutic approaches, such as individualized probiotic regimens designed to help the gut heal itself.

In summary, the current status of celiac disease research is distinguished by a multimodal approach that includes genetics, diagnosis, and the complex interrelationships between celiac disease and other medical disorders. These discoveries not only deepen our knowledge of the illness but also open the door to more focused and successful treatment approaches.

Prospective Developments and Innovations:

Celiac disease sufferers now have hope thanks to encouraging developments and discoveries in the fight against the difficult illness in recent years. The investigation of non-dietary therapeutic possibilities is one noteworthy development. Strict adherence to a gluten-free diet is the traditional approach to management, however, current research is looking into alternate therapeutic options. Clinical trials are demonstrating the potential of enzyme therapy aimed at breaking down gluten in the digestive tract. If these enzymes are shown to be beneficial, they may provide people with celiac disease with more food options.

Moreover, immunotherapy has become a ground-breaking method. Research is being done on vaccines and immunomodulatory medications that target the immune response to gluten. By desensitizing the immune system, these therapies let people tolerate gluten without experiencing negative side effects. Early-phase clinical trial preliminary results are promising and suggest that the paradigm for celiac disease therapy may change.

The creation of gadgets that can detect gluten is another significant advancement. With the introduction of portable and easily navigable gadgets that can identify gluten in food, people with celiac disease may now make educated dietary decisions. These gadgets are revolutionary because they offer a level of control that goes beyond carefully reading labels and examining ingredients.

Furthermore, the importance of patient-centered care and support is rising. With the proliferation of online forums, mobile apps, and online communities devoted to celiac disease, people now have a place to talk about their experiences, get trustworthy information, and get advice from professionals.

The individuals impacted by celiac disease are feeling more empowered and part of a community thanks to this integrated network.

In conclusion, there have been encouraging developments in non-dietary therapies, immunotherapy, gluten detection technology, and improved patient support systems that are changing the face of celiac disease treatment. These discoveries represent a paradigm shift in the treatment of celiac disease and have the potential to greatly enhance the lives of those afflicted with this autoimmune condition.

Taking Part in Clinical Research:

Taking part in clinical studies is essential to improving our knowledge of and ability to treat celiac disease. New treatments, diagnostic techniques, and interventions are developed and evaluated primarily through clinical trials. Participating in clinical trials allows people with celiac disease to further their understanding of the illness and gain access to novel therapies before they are generally distributed.

Access to cutting-edge therapy techniques is one alluring feature of taking part in clinical trials. These studies frequently assess immunotherapies, enzyme treatments, and experimental medications, giving participants a chance to personally witness the effectiveness and safety of novel interventions. Those who have not found the best relief from conventional gluten-free treatment may benefit most from this early exposure.

Moreover, taking part in clinical studies offers people with celiac disease a special chance to help create more precise diagnostic instruments.

To improve the accuracy and speed of celiac disease diagnosis, trials frequently evaluate novel biomarkers, genetic tests, or imaging modalities. Participants have a significant influence on how celiac disease diagnosis methods will develop in the future by voluntarily participating in these studies.

Participating in clinical trials is advantageous for each participant individually as well as for the greater scientific community, which helps to better understand the illness. Researchers can learn more about the subtleties of celiac disease, its underlying mechanisms, and the varying reactions to various treatments thanks to the data collected by these trials. This body of knowledge is essential for improving currently available treatments and creating fresh plans for controlling and eventually curing celiac disease.

Nonetheless, it's crucial to approach taking part in clinical trials thoughtfully. Those who are thinking about participating should be fully aware of the trial's possible dangers and advantages, talk to their medical professionals about it, and make decisions based on their own set of circumstances.

In summary, taking part in clinical trials is an excellent and significant method for people with celiac disease to influence the direction of future celiac disease therapy, obtain access to cutting-edge medicines, and support scientific advances. This cooperative effort between participants and researchers is essential to advancing the development of more accessible, individualized, and successful treatments for people with celiac disease.

CHAPTER TEN

COMMUNITY SUPPORT AND ADVOCACY
Raising Awareness of Celiac Disease:

Promoting compassion and empathy in communities begins with raising awareness of celiac disease. Often, celiac disease is misdiagnosed or misinterpreted, causing needless misery for people who are afflicted. Spreading proper knowledge about celiac disease, its symptoms, and the gluten-free diet that sufferers must follow are all part of the advocacy for celiac awareness.

Numerous platforms, including social media, neighborhood gatherings, and instructional seminars, can be used to start educational initiatives. Working together with nutritionists and medical specialists to develop easily understood tools will enable people to identify the symptoms of Celiac disease and seek an appropriate diagnosis and course of treatment.

Busting myths and false beliefs about celiac disease is a crucial part of raising awareness. Many individuals may be unaware of how serious the illness is or how gluten might affect those who have celiac disease. By using first-person accounts and testimonies, it is possible to personalize the experiences of people with celiac disease and promote empathy and understanding. Through public outreach initiatives, written pieces, and neighborhood gatherings, we can better educate the public and foster a supportive environment for those who suffer from celiac disease.

Joining Support Groups for Celiacs:

Support groups are essential for developing a feeling of camaraderie and mutual understanding among people with celiac disease. Those who join these organizations get access to a forum where they may interact, trade insightful knowledge, and discuss experiences. These support groups can provide practical advice on negotiating social and everyday obstacles related to celiac disease, as well as emotional support and guidance on managing a gluten-free lifestyle. Furthermore, support groups frequently plan workshops, webinars, and other activities that advance information sharing and the growth of a robust support system.

Taking part in support groups for people with celiac disease helps them feel less alone and more like part of the community. It enables people to celebrate victories, exchange coping mechanisms, and gain insight from one another's experiences. Additionally, these organizations can act as community advocates, banding together to increase awareness and impact favorable changes in laws and public opinion. Through active participation in Celiac support groups, those impacted by the illness can strengthen the bonds within the community and make their voices heard in the larger advocacy space.

Promoting Changes in Policy:

One of the most important aspects of the larger initiative to enhance the lives of people with celiac disease is advocating for changes in legislation.

The well-being of individuals impacted by policies at many levels, such as healthcare, education, and food labeling, can be greatly impacted. To guarantee that the requirements of the celiac community are acknowledged and taken into consideration throughout the formulation and execution of policy, legislators, medical professionals, and pertinent organizations must be involved.

The fight for better guidelines for gluten-free labeling is one of the main advocacy areas. By assisting people with Celiac disease in making educated food choices, clear and accurate labeling lowers the possibility of unintentional gluten intake. Furthermore, promoting greater accessibility to gluten-free options in public areas, educational institutions, and medical facilities is essential for promoting inclusivity.

Furthermore, promoting more money for celiac disease research can help develop new methods of diagnosis, care, and ultimately, a cure. Through joint efforts with other advocacy groups, medical experts, and researchers, the Celiac community's combined voice can effect legislative changes that improve the quality of life for individuals living with the condition. In addition to resolving the current issues, the advocacy for legislative reforms aims to foster a welcoming and accommodating environment for future generations of celiac disease sufferers.

CHAPTER ELEVEN

OVERCOMING CELIAC DISEASE TO SUCCEED
Techniques for Living a Happy and Healthful Life

Living with celiac disease necessitates a multimodal strategy to maintain social and emotional as well as physical well-being. Keeping to a rigorous gluten-free diet is one of the main methods for living well after being diagnosed with celiac disease.

In people with celiac disease, gluten—which is present in wheat, barley, and rye—sets off immunological reactions that result in inflammation and minor intestinal damage. Patients can control their symptoms and encourage healing by removing gluten from their diet. But leading a gluten-free lifestyle is more than just avoiding specific foods; it also calls for careful label reading, inventive cooking, and frequently the assistance of dietitians and medical professionals.

Education and awareness are also essential for those with celiac disease to lead healthy and productive lives. Patients who are aware of their condition are better equipped to make decisions regarding their health. This entails keeping up with gluten-free substitutes, figuring out how to handle food-related social settings, and identifying gluten-containing hidden sources. Education benefits not only the individual but also the community at large, friends, and family.

Establishing a conducive atmosphere greatly enhances the general welfare of individuals with celiac disease by promoting comprehension and reducing the obstacles they might encounter in all facets of their lives.

Adopting a holistic perspective on health is essential. Due to the frequent correlation between celiac disease and other autoimmune disorders, routine medical examinations and surveillance for linked health problems are crucial. Using stress-reduction strategies, exercising frequently, and getting enough sleep are all essential parts of this comprehensive approach. Since managing a chronic condition can have a substantial psychological impact, mental health is something that should not be disregarded. Getting help from online communities, support groups, or mental health specialists can help manage the emotional difficulties brought on by celiac disease.

Honoring Achievements

To promote motivation, hope, and a sense of community among those living with celiac disease, it is essential to highlight success stories. These success tales frequently feature people who have triumphed over various celiac disease-related obstacles and come out stronger on the inside as well as the outside. Telling these tales serves as a monument to the tenacity of those with celiac disease as well as a source of inspiration.

Within the celiac community, there are many different kinds of success stories. Some people might talk about how they successfully followed a gluten-free diet and how it improved their quality of life and health. Others might concentrate on their accomplishments, such as controlling the illness while achieving professional success, engaging in physical pursuits, or interacting confidently in social circumstances.

Beyond personal achievements, community projects, awareness campaigns, and breakthroughs in celiac disease research are all worthy of celebration. It is crucial to acknowledge the work done by researchers, advocacy organizations, and medical professionals who advance our knowledge of and ability to treat celiac disease. By showcasing these accomplishments, the larger community is educated, involved, and inspired to keep encouraging and supporting people who are impacted by celiac disease.

Outlook for Celiac Patients in the Future

Prospects for celiac disease patients appear bright, with more options for diagnosis, treatment, and overall quality of life expected as long as medical science and technology continue to progress. To gain a deeper understanding of the fundamental causes of celiac disease, researchers are experimenting with novel approaches that could lead to the development of targeted treatments and individualized treatment regimens. This includes looking into potential biomarkers that could support early identification and intervention, the gut microbiome, and genetic variables.

Regarding therapy, new drugs and treatments are being investigated in current clinical studies to control the symptoms of celiac disease and encourage intestine repair. These developments might provide options for people who find it difficult to follow a gluten-free diet precisely or who still have symptoms after making dietary changes.

Future developments in gluten detection techniques could also make it simpler for people to recognize and steer clear of gluten-containing goods. This can lessen the social obstacles that people with celiac disease frequently experience by fostering a more accepting and understanding society in conjunction with raising awareness and educating the public.

A more understanding and accommodating world for celiac patients is also being shaped by continuous work in the areas of patient advocacy and support. Growing awareness is likely to lead to better funding for research, easier access to gluten-free products, and stronger support systems, all of which will benefit those living with and beyond celiac disease in the long run.

www.ingramcontent.com/pod-product-compliance
Lightning Source LLC
Chambersburg PA
CBHW050742260726

48661CB00001B/374